TAI CHI AS THERAPEUTIC MEDICINE

Embodied Regulation for Chronic Illness, Stability, and Neurodegenerative Care

BY
MOSHE PITCHON

Editorial & Copyright Page
Tai Chi as Therapeutic Medicine
Embodied Regulation for Chronic Illness, Aging, and Neurological Care
© 2026 by **Moshe (Maurice) Pitchon**
All rights reserved.
No part of this book may be reproduced, stored in a retrieval system, or transmitted in any form or by any means—electronic, mechanical, photocopying, recording, or otherwise—without the prior written permission of the publisher, except for brief quotations in reviews or scholarly works.
Author
Moshe (Maurice) Pitchon
Publisher
TCHWUSA'
[Miami-Florida-Usa]
TCHWUSA.com
ISBN Information
ISBN 978- ISBN: 979-8-9925712-9-5
(Paperback)
ISBN ISBN: 979-8-9925712-8-8 (eBook)
Editorial Disclaimer
This book is intended for educational and informational purposes only. It does not provide medical advice, diagnosis, or treatment. The practices described herein are not a substitute for professional medical care. Readers should consult qualified healthcare providers regarding any medical condition or before beginning any new health or movement program.
The author and publisher disclaim responsibility for any adverse effects resulting directly or indirectly from the use or application of the information contained in this book.

Scope of Practice Notice
Tai Chi instructors and programs discussed in this book operate within a non-medical scope of practice. They do not diagnose conditions, prescribe treatments, or offer prognostic claims. All therapeutic applications described are intended to complement—not replace—medical care.
Printed in the United States of America
First edition

Dedication

This book is dedicated to my Tai Chi Sifu, **Rafael Rivero**, whose mastery, devotion to the art, and inspiring presence have shaped my understanding of practice and purpose. For his teaching and his example, I remain deeply grateful.

It is also dedicated to the memory of my karate sensei, **Michihiza Itaya**, who, more than six decades ago, first opened for me the doors to the Far Eastern wisdom of the body and the discipline through which it is formed.

Contents

Preface: Why This Book Was Written 7
Introduction: Why Tai Chi Must Be Understood as Medicine-in-Movement   9

PART I: FOUNDATIONS 11
Chapter One: Tai Chi as Embodied Chinese Medicine 13
Chapter Two: Why Western Medicine Took Notice 19

PART II: CORE THERAPEUTIC FUNCTIONS 25
Chapter Three: Stability, Balance, and Fall Prevention 27
Chapter Four: Parkinson's Disease: Movement Without Force 33
Chapter Five: Arthritis and Rheumatism: Motion Without Aggression 39

PART III: INTEGRATION INTO CARE SETTINGS 45
Chapter Six: Respiratory Regulation, Sleep, and Apnea 47
Chapter Seven: Tai Chi in Clinical and Residential Environments 53
Chapter Eight: Designing Therapeutic Tai Chi Programs 59

PART IV: THE FUTURE OF THERAPEUTIC TAI CHI 65
Chapter Nine: From Complementary to Essential 67
Chapter Ten: Tai Chi as a Medical Culture, Not a Technique 73

Book Conclusion 77
Postscript 79

APPENDICES 83
Appendix A : Program Safety Checklist 85
Appendix B : Instructor Competency Framework 87
Appendix C 89
Appendix D: Modern Wellness Tai Chi Sequence Vocabulary 91
Bibliography 93

Preface

Why This Book Was Written

This book was written slowly.

Not because Tai Chi resists explanation, but because the questions it raises cannot be answered quickly. They concern how human beings live with chronic limitation, how medicine responds when cure is no longer the horizon, and how movement can become a site of responsibility rather than performance.

I did not begin this work to promote Tai Chi, nor to defend Chinese Medicine against modern science. I began it after observing a recurring pattern across clinical, residential, and community settings: people were surviving longer, but living with less confidence in their bodies. Falls, fear of movement, chronic pain, neurological instability, and respiratory dysregulation were not isolated problems—they were signs of a deeper breakdown in regulation.

Tai Chi appeared repeatedly in this landscape, not as a miracle solution, but as something quietly effective. It was tolerated where other programs failed. It was sustained where interventions were abandoned. It restored participation where withdrawal had become the norm.

This book is an attempt to explain why.

Introduction

Why Tai Chi Must Be Understood as Medicine-in-Movement

Modern medicine has achieved extraordinary success in treating acute illness. Yet its greatest challenge today lies elsewhere: in chronic conditions that do not resolve, fluctuate unpredictably, and demand long-term engagement rather than decisive intervention.

In these conditions—Parkinson's disease, arthritis, balance disorders, sleep dysregulation, neurodegenerative decline—the central question is no longer *How do we cure?* but *How do we support life within limitation?*

Tai Chi enters this question not as an alternative to medicine, but as a response to what medicine leaves unfinished. Rooted in Chinese Medicine's emphasis on balance, continuity, and regulation, Tai Chi translates these principles into embodied practice. It does not treat disease directly. It trains the conditions under which regulation becomes possible.

Western medicine did not adopt Tai Chi out of cultural curiosity. It adopted it because it worked—quietly, consistently, and where other interventions reached their limits.

This book develops that story.

PART I:
FOUNDATIONS

Chapter One

Tai Chi as Embodied Chinese Medicine

Chinese Medicine as Pattern Recognition, Not Disease Labeling

Chinese Medicine does not begin with disease. It begins with **patterns**—patterns of tension and release, excess and deficiency, stagnation and flow.

Its diagnostic categories do not ask first *what illness a person has*, but *how regulation has broken down*. Symptoms are not isolated malfunctions; they are expressions of systemic imbalance.

This orientation is fundamentally different from the Western biomedical model, which tends to localize pathology in organs, tissues, or biochemical processes. While Western medicine excels at acute intervention—surgery, pharmacology, emergency care—it often struggles with conditions that unfold over time, fluctuate in severity, and resist definitive resolution. Chronic illness, neurodegeneration, and age-related functional decline expose this limitation with particular clarity.

Chinese Medicine, by contrast, has always been a medicine of **continuity rather than interruption**. Its concern is not the eradication of symptoms, but the restoration of conditions under which the organism can regulate itself more effectively. Diagnosis names patterns; therapy seeks to reorganize them.

Tai Chi emerges from this same medical worldview.

From Diagnosis to Regulation: Why Movement Matters

Most people encounter Chinese Medicine through acupuncture, herbal prescriptions, or dietary recommendations. These modalities are often understood as *treatments applied to the body*. Tai Chi operates differently. It does not apply medicine to the organism; it *trains the organism to reorganize itself*.

This distinction is crucial.

Where acupuncture intervenes at specific points and herbs modulate internal chemistry, Tai Chi engages the *entire regulatory system simultaneously*. Posture, breath, attention, balance, and timing are not treated separately; they are integrated through slow, continuous movement. The practitioner does not receive treatment passively but participates actively in the process of regulation.

In this sense, Tai Chi functions as *diagnosis-in-motion*. Every shift of weight reveals balance strategies. Every transition exposes coordination patterns. Tension, collapse, hesitation, or rigidity are not abstract concepts; they are experienced directly and corrected through practice. The body learns—not intellectually, but somatically—how imbalance feels and how balance is restored.

This is why Tai Chi cannot be reduced to exercise.

Qi, Balance, and Functional Integration (Without Mysticism)

In Chinese Medicine, *qi* names the capacity for coordinated function. It is not a substance, nor a metaphorical energy divorced from physiology. It refers to **the ability of systems to communicate, adapt, and respond**. When qi is described as "stagnant" or "deficient," what is being named is not a mystical force, but a loss of coordination, timing, or resilience.

Tai Chi trains qi by training **functional integration**.

Slow movement amplifies feedback. Continuous transitions eliminate abrupt force. Weight transfer teaches the nervous system how to distribute load without strain. Attention synchronizes intention and action. Breath anchors movement in rhythm rather than effort. Together, these elements cultivate balance not as a static posture, but as a **dynamic capacity**.

From a modern perspective, this corresponds to improvements in proprioception, neuromuscular coordination, autonomic regulation, and postural reflexes. Tai Chi strengthens the system not by pushing it to extremes, but by refining its internal communication.

The language differs; the function does not.

Tai Chi as Medical Amplification, Not Exercise

It is tempting—especially in Western contexts—to frame Tai Chi as a "gentle exercise" or a "mind-body activity." While these descriptions are not entirely wrong, they are deeply insufficient. Exercise focuses on exertion, repetition, and performance metrics. Tai Chi focuses on **organization, continuity, and adaptability**.

Exercise trains muscles.

Tai Chi trains **coordination**.

Exercise isolates variables.

Tai Chi integrates systems.

Exercise often emphasizes effort.

Tai Chi emphasizes efficiency.

This distinction explains why Tai Chi remains effective even when participants are frail, cognitively impaired, or physically limited. The practice does not demand strength before coordination; it cultivates coordination as the foundation from which strength may gradually emerge.

Seen this way, Tai Chi is best understood as an **amplification of Chinese Medicine's logic**, translated into embodied practice. It does not replace acupuncture or herbal therapy; it extends their underlying principles into daily movement. It teaches the body to become an active participant in its own regulation.

Why This Framework Translates Across Cultures

One of the most remarkable aspects of Tai Chi's modern therapeutic adoption is its success outside its original cultural context. Western clinicians and researchers did not embrace Tai Chi because they accepted Chinese cosmology. They embraced it because **it worked**.

Tai Chi's medical logic translates because it addresses universal human problems:

- Loss of balance
- Decline in coordination
- Chronic pain
- Neurological instability
- Respiratory dysregulation
- Fear of movement
- Reduced confidence in the body

These are not culturally specific conditions. They are features of aging, illness, and stress across societies.

By reframing Tai Chi as **medicine embodied rather than explained**, it becomes possible to integrate it into clinical settings without requiring belief, ideology, or philosophical conversion. What is required is only attention to function, safety, and adaptation.

This book proceeds from that premise.

Tai Chi is not an alternative to medicine.

It is **a medical intelligence expressed through movement**.

In the chapters that follow, we will see why Western medicine—faced with the growing burden of chronic illness—eventually recognized this fact, and how Tai Chi came to occupy a legitimate place in therapeutic research and care.

Chapter Summary

Tai Chi emerges from the same regulatory logic as Chinese Medicine, but expresses that logic through continuous movement rather than discrete intervention. By training coordination, balance, breath, and attention simultaneously, it amplifies the body's capacity for self-regulation. This functional orientation—not cultural mysticism—explains why Tai Chi translates effectively into modern therapeutic contexts.

Chapter Two

Why Western Medicine Took Notice

The Rise of Chronic Illness and Aging Populations

For much of the twentieth century, Western medicine was shaped by a model of acute intervention. Infection, trauma, and discrete pathological events dominated medical practice. The physician intervened, the condition resolved, and care concluded. This model proved extraordinarily effective—and remains indispensable.

Yet over time, the epidemiological landscape shifted.

Chronic illnesses, neurodegenerative disorders, autoimmune conditions, and age-related functional decline became the dominant medical challenges of advanced societies. These conditions do not resolve through single interventions. They unfold gradually, fluctuate unpredictably, and often persist despite optimal pharmacological management. The success of modern medicine in extending life expectancy paradoxically intensified this problem: more people were living longer with conditions that medicine could manage, but not cure.

This shift forced a reckoning. Western healthcare systems increasingly confronted a population whose primary needs were not survival, but *function, stability, autonomy, and quality of life*.

It is within this context—not through philosophical curiosity—that

Tai Chi entered Western medical attention.

Where Pharmacology Reaches Its Limits

Pharmacological treatment remains essential in the management of chronic disease. Medications reduce symptoms, slow progression, and improve survival. Yet they rarely restore lost function on their own. Moreover, long-term medication use carries cumulative risks: side effects, interactions, tolerance, and diminished efficacy over time.

In conditions such as Parkinson's disease, arthritis, balance disorders, sleep dysregulation, and respiratory impairment, medication addresses biochemical pathways but leaves **functional integration largely untouched**. A patient may experience symptom relief without regaining confidence in movement, coordination, or bodily awareness. Fear of falling, avoidance of motion, and progressive deconditioning often follow.

Clinicians increasingly recognized a gap between what medicine could *control* and what patients needed in order to *live well*. That gap was not primarily biochemical. It was functional.

Tai Chi emerged as one of several non-pharmacological approaches investigated to address this unmet need.

The Search for Low-Risk, Scalable Interventions

As healthcare systems grappled with rising costs, aging populations, and workforce constraints, the search intensified for interventions that were:

- Low risk
- Non-invasive
- Cost-effective
- Scalable across large populations

- Adaptable to varying levels of ability
- Sustainable over long periods

Tai Chi met these criteria in ways few interventions could.

Unlike high-intensity exercise programs, Tai Chi required no specialized equipment, minimal space, and could be practiced standing, seated, or with assistance. Injury risk was low. Dropout rates were comparatively modest. Most importantly, participants were often willing to continue practicing beyond formal study periods, suggesting long-term viability.

These practical advantages mattered. But they alone would not have been sufficient to attract sustained scientific interest.

What ultimately drew attention were **measurable outcomes**.

Why Tai Chi Fit Clinical Criteria

When Western researchers began studying Tai Chi, they did not frame it as a cultural artifact. They approached it as a **functional intervention**. The questions were pragmatic:

- Does it reduce falls?
- Does it improve gait and balance?
- Does it enhance motor control?
- Does it reduce pain?
- Does it improve sleep and respiratory regulation?
- Does it enhance confidence and reduce fear of movement?

Across diverse populations and study designs, Tai Chi repeatedly demonstrated modest but consistent benefits in precisely these domains. Importantly, these benefits often appeared **where other interventions showed diminishing returns**—particularly in older adults and individuals with chronic neurological or musculoskeletal conditions.

Tai Chi's effectiveness was not dramatic in the sense of acute cures.

Its strength lay in **incremental functional improvement**, maintained over time. From a medical perspective, this is precisely the kind of intervention chronic care requires.

Equally significant was what Tai Chi did *not* do: it did not overwhelm compromised systems. It did not demand strength before coordination. It did not impose speed where timing was already impaired. It respected the limits of the organism while gently reorganizing how those limits were negotiated.

How Research Followed Outcomes, Not Philosophy

Western medical research did not begin by attempting to validate Chinese medical theory. It began by observing results. Balance improved. Falls decreased. Gait stabilized. Pain lessened. Sleep quality improved. Participants reported greater confidence in movement and reduced fear.

Only afterward did researchers begin asking *why*.

Neuroscience provided part of the explanation: enhanced proprioception, improved motor planning, increased cortical engagement, and refined postural reflexes. Physiology contributed another layer: improved respiratory efficiency, autonomic regulation, and circulation. Psychology added still another: reduced anxiety, increased self-efficacy, and renewed trust in the body.

None of these explanations required acceptance of traditional Chinese cosmology. Yet all of them were fully compatible with Chinese Medicine's emphasis on regulation, balance, and integration.

In this way, Tai Chi crossed a cultural boundary not by translating its language, but by demonstrating its function.

From Marginal Practice to Therapeutic Category

Over time, Tai Chi moved from the margins of "complementary and alternative medicine" toward a more precise classification: **a therapeutic movement practice with regulatory effects**. It came to be studied alongside physical therapy, balance training, and neurological rehabilitation—sometimes compared, sometimes integrated.

What distinguished Tai Chi was not that it replaced these modalities, but that it addressed dimensions they often left underdeveloped: continuity, internal coordination, and attentional engagement. Tai Chi did not merely strengthen muscles or retrain specific movements; it *reeducated the organism's relationship to movement itself.*

This distinction matters profoundly in chronic illness, where fear, hesitation, and loss of confidence often accelerate decline more than pathology alone.

Why Tai Chi Continues to Attract Medical Interest

Tai Chi continues to attract research interest because it sits at a rare intersection:

- It is ancient but adaptable
- Structured yet flexible
- Gentle yet neurologically demanding
- Simple in appearance, complex in effect

As healthcare systems increasingly prioritize prevention, functional independence, and quality of life, Tai Chi's relevance grows rather than diminishes. It offers a way to work with the body's regulatory capacities rather than against them.

In doing so, it answers a question modern medicine increasingly asks but rarely articulates clearly:

How can we help people live well with conditions that cannot be

cured?

Chapter Summary

Western medicine's interest in Tai Chi did not arise from cultural fascination, but from clinical necessity. Faced with chronic illness, aging populations, and the limits of pharmacological intervention, researchers sought low-risk, scalable approaches that improved function rather than merely controlled symptoms. Tai Chi met these needs by enhancing coordination, balance, and regulatory capacity—demonstrating measurable outcomes without imposing excessive strain. Its adoption reflects a broader shift toward therapies that support ongoing regulation rather than episodic intervention.

PART II:
CORE THERAPEUTIC FUNCTIONS

(Each chapter follows the same internal logic for consistency and credibility)

Chapter Three

Stability, Balance, and Fall Prevention

Why Falls Are a Medical Emergency in Aging

Falls are among the most serious and underestimated threats to health in older adults. They are not merely accidents; they are often the first visible sign of declining neurological integration, postural control, and confidence in movement. A single fall can trigger a cascade of consequences—fracture, hospitalization, loss of independence, institutionalization, and increased mortality.

Equally important, the *fear of falling* frequently proves more disabling than the fall itself. Once confidence in balance erodes, individuals restrict movement, reduce activity, and withdraw from daily tasks. This self-protective response accelerates deconditioning, weakens postural reflexes, and paradoxically increases fall risk.

From a medical standpoint, falls represent a failure of **regulation**, not strength alone. Muscles may still function, vision may remain intact, and reflexes may be present, yet the system as a whole fails to coordinate rapidly enough to maintain stability during transitions. This is precisely where Tai Chi operates most effectively.

Balance as a Neurological Function

Balance is often misunderstood as a mechanical issue—something solved by strengthening legs or improving flexibility. In reality, balance is a **complex neurological process** involving continuous integration of sensory input, motor planning, and anticipatory adjustment.

Maintaining stability requires:

- Proprioceptive awareness (knowing where the body is in space)
- Vestibular processing (orientation and equilibrium)
- Visual input
- Postural reflexes
- Timing and coordination between upper and lower body
- Confidence and attentional focus

Disruption in any one of these components can destabilize the entire system. Aging, neurological disease, medication effects, and prolonged inactivity all degrade this integration over time.

Tai Chi addresses balance not by isolating components, but by **retraining their cooperation**.

Tai Chi and Weight Transfer

At the heart of Tai Chi lies a deceptively simple action: **controlled weight transfer**. Every movement requires the practitioner to shift weight from one leg to the other, often slowly, deliberately, and without external support.

This process accomplishes several therapeutic goals simultaneously:

- It retrains the nervous system to recognize load changes
- It improves timing between intention and execution
- It reduces reliance on rigid bracing strategies
- It restores trust in single-leg support
- It strengthens stabilizing muscles without impact

Unlike conventional balance exercises, Tai Chi does not train balance in static positions alone. It emphasizes **transitional stability**—the ability to remain organized while moving from one state to another. Most falls occur not while standing still, but during transitions: turning, reaching, stepping, or changing direction.

Tai Chi practices these moments continuously.

Proprioception, Rooting, and Postural Reflexes

In Chinese Medicine, stability is often described through the metaphor of "rooting"—the body's ability to remain connected to the ground while remaining mobile above it. Stripped of metaphor, this refers to **efficient ground reaction force management**.

Tai Chi enhances proprioception by:

- Slowing movement enough to amplify sensory feedback
- Encouraging awareness of pressure through the feet
- Aligning joints to distribute load efficiently
- Reducing unnecessary muscular tension

As proprioceptive clarity improves, postural reflexes become more responsive. Instead of reacting late with exaggerated corrections, the body begins to anticipate imbalance and adjust subtly. This anticipatory control is crucial for fall prevention.

Importantly, Tai Chi cultivates these reflexes without provoking anxiety. Movements are slow, predictable, and reversible. Participants are not pushed to the edge of their capacity; they are invited to **explore it safely**.

Research Findings: Functional Outcomes

Across numerous studies involving older adults and individuals with balance impairments, Tai Chi has been associated with:

- Reduced incidence of falls
- Improved gait speed and stride consistency
- Enhanced single-leg stance time
- Improved postural control
- Reduced fear of falling
- Increased confidence in movement

While effect sizes vary, the consistency of these findings across populations and settings is notable. Tai Chi rarely produces dramatic short-term changes. Instead, it delivers **reliable, cumulative improvements** in functional stability.

From a clinical perspective, this is precisely the outcome that matters most. Preventing even a modest percentage of falls translates into substantial reductions in injury, hospitalization, and long-term care costs—along with immeasurable benefits to dignity and independence.

Therapeutic Adaptations: Standing, Seated, and Assisted Practice

One of Tai Chi's greatest strengths as a therapeutic modality is its adaptability. Balance training does not require that participants begin in a standing position. In fact, for individuals with severe instability, seated practice may be both safer and more effective initially.

Standing practice emphasizes:
- Weight transfer
- Single-leg loading
- Postural alignment
- Transitional control

Seated practice emphasizes:
- Trunk stability
- Pelvic orientation
- Upper-lower body coordination

- Proprioceptive awareness without fall risk

Assisted practice—using chairs, bars, or light support—allows individuals to explore balance transitions while maintaining a margin of safety.

Crucially, therapeutic Tai Chi does not follow a fixed progression schedule. Advancement depends on **functional readiness**, not time spent practicing. This individualized pacing distinguishes therapeutic Tai Chi from standardized exercise protocols.

Restoring Confidence in Movement

Perhaps the most overlooked benefit of Tai Chi in fall prevention is psychological rather than mechanical. Through repeated, successful experiences of controlled movement, participants gradually rebuild **trust in their bodies**.

Confidence reduces hesitation. Reduced hesitation improves timing. Improved timing reduces falls.

This virtuous cycle cannot be achieved through instruction alone. It must be **experienced**. Tai Chi provides a structured environment in which such experience becomes possible.

Chapter Summary

Falls result from failures of coordination, timing, and confidence—not strength alone. Tai Chi addresses balance as a neurological and regulatory function by retraining weight transfer, proprioception, and postural reflexes through slow, continuous movement. Its emphasis on transitional stability, adaptability, and safety makes it particularly effective for older adults and individuals at risk of falling. By restoring both functional integration and confidence in movement, Tai Chi reduces fall risk while supporting independence and quality of life.

Chapter Four

Parkinson's Disease: Movement Without Force

Parkinson's Beyond Tremor

Parkinson's disease is often publicly associated with tremor. Clinically, however, tremor is only one—and not always the most disabling—manifestation of a far more complex disorder. Parkinson's fundamentally disrupts *the timing, initiation, and coordination of movement.* Patients frequently describe feeling as though the intention to move and the body's ability to respond have fallen out of sync.

Bradykinesia, rigidity, postural instability, freezing of gait, and reduced facial and gestural expressiveness all reflect this deeper disruption. Movements that were once automatic now require conscious effort. Transitions—standing up, turning, initiating a step—become precarious. Over time, fear of freezing or falling further constrains movement, compounding physical decline with psychological withdrawal.

Medication can mitigate symptoms, particularly in early and mid stages of the disease. Yet even when pharmacological management is optimized, many patients continue to struggle with coordination, balance, and confidence. Parkinson's reveals with particular clarity the limits of symptom control when **functional integration itself is impaired**.

It is precisely within this space that Tai Chi has attracted sustained therapeutic interest.

Timing, Initiation, and Motor Planning

At its core, Parkinson's disease disrupts the brain's ability to initiate and smoothly sequence movement. Actions that once flowed automatically must be consciously assembled, step by step. This makes speed a liability rather than an asset. Rapid or forceful movement often exacerbates instability, increases freezing episodes, and undermines confidence.

Tai Chi inverts this dynamic.

By slowing movement to a deliberate, continuous pace, Tai Chi reduces the neurological demand for rapid initiation. Each action unfolds gradually, allowing intention, perception, and execution to remain aligned. The practitioner is not required to "react" quickly, but to *remain present throughout the movement's entire trajectory.*

This sustained attentional engagement supports motor planning rather than bypassing it. Movements are initiated gently, completed fully, and transitioned smoothly—qualities that are often compromised in Parkinson's but remain trainable.

Tai Chi's Slow-Speed Neurological Recalibration

Tai Chi's defining characteristic—slow, continuous movement—is not an aesthetic choice. It is a neurological strategy.

Slow speed:

- Enhances sensory feedback
- Allows time for postural adjustment
- Reduces reliance on reflexive bracing
- Supports anticipatory control
- Minimizes abrupt motor commands

For individuals with Parkinson's, this creates a safer environment in which movement can be explored without triggering freezing or loss of balance. Because movements are reversible and non-ballistic, errors do not escalate into crises. This lowers anxiety and encourages continued participation.

Over time, repeated exposure to controlled movement sequences appears to support **recalibration of motor timing**. While Tai Chi does not alter the underlying pathology of Parkinson's disease, it can improve how the nervous system works *with* that pathology rather than constantly struggling against it.

Mind–Movement Coupling

One of the most debilitating aspects of Parkinson's is the fragmentation between intention and action. Tai Chi directly addresses this by requiring continuous coupling between attention and movement.

In Tai Chi:

- Attention leads movement
- Movement feeds back into attention
- Breath anchors both

This closed loop reinforces agency. The practitioner does not simply perform movements; they *inhabit* them. For Parkinson's patients, this sense of agency is therapeutically significant. It counteracts the feeling that the body has become unreliable or alien.

Unlike repetitive exercise routines, Tai Chi sequences demand moment-to-moment awareness. Each shift of weight, rotation of the torso, and placement of the foot requires conscious participation. This engagement appears to support neural pathways involved in coordination and postural control, even in the presence of neurodegenerative change.

Research Outcomes in Parkinson's Disease

Across multiple clinical studies, Tai Chi has been associated with improvements in:

- Postural stability
- Gait control
- Functional mobility
- Balance confidence
- Reduction in fall frequency
- Overall quality of life

Importantly, Tai Chi has often compared favorably to resistance training and stretching in balance-related outcomes, particularly in reducing falls and improving functional reach. These findings suggest that Tai Chi's strength lies not in building force, but in refining **control, timing, and adaptability**.

As with other chronic conditions, improvements are typically modest but consistent. Tai Chi is not a cure. Its value lies in slowing functional decline, preserving independence, and improving daily experience.

From a therapeutic standpoint, these are decisive outcomes.

Safety and Adaptation Principles

Therapeutic Tai Chi for Parkinson's disease must prioritize safety, adaptability, and respect for fluctuating capacity. Symptoms vary not only between individuals, but within the same individual across days and even hours.

Key principles include:

- Avoiding speed and force
- Emphasizing stable transitions
- Allowing seated or supported practice when needed
- Reducing cognitive overload

- Maintaining predictable movement patterns
- Encouraging rest without framing it as failure

Seated Tai Chi can be particularly effective in advanced stages, allowing patients to engage trunk rotation, weight shifting, and coordinated arm movements without fall risk. Assisted standing practice may be introduced gradually, based on confidence rather than chronological progression.

Therapeutic success depends less on technical precision than on **maintaining continuity of engagement**.

Preserving Dignity and Agency

Beyond measurable motor outcomes, Tai Chi offers something of equal importance to individuals living with Parkinson's disease: a way to move without being constantly reminded of limitation.

Because Tai Chi emphasizes quality over quantity and coherence over performance, participants are not judged against external standards. Progress is internal, experiential, and individualized. This preserves dignity in a condition that often erodes it.

Tai Chi does not ask Parkinson's patients to overcome their condition. It teaches them how to **inhabit their bodies more fully within it**.

Chapter Summary

Parkinson's disease disrupts movement at the level of timing, initiation, and coordination rather than strength alone. Tai Chi addresses these challenges by slowing movement, enhancing sensory feedback, and reinforcing mind–movement coupling. Through continuous, controlled transitions, Tai Chi supports postural stability, reduces fall risk, and restores confidence in movement. While it does not alter disease progression, it offers a safe, adaptable means of preserving function, agency, and quality of life.

Chapter Five

Arthritis and Rheumatism: Motion Without Aggression

Why "Exercise" Often Fails Arthritis Patients

For individuals living with arthritis and rheumatic conditions, movement is frequently framed as a paradox. On one hand, inactivity worsens stiffness, weakness, and pain. On the other, conventional exercise often exacerbates symptoms, reinforces fear, and leads to repeated cycles of overexertion followed by withdrawal.

Many exercise programs emphasize intensity, repetition, and muscular load. While these approaches may benefit healthy individuals, they can be counterproductive for those whose joints are inflamed, structurally compromised, or chronically sensitive. Pain becomes a signal to stop, and movement is associated with damage rather than healing.

Over time, this dynamic foster **movement avoidance**, loss of joint mobility, and progressive deconditioning. The problem is not that people with arthritis cannot move, but that they are often asked to move in ways that **ignore the regulatory limits of their condition**.

Tai Chi offers a fundamentally different approach.

Joint Health as Dynamic Circulation

From the perspective of Chinese Medicine, pain and stiffness are signs of impaired circulation and disrupted coordination. Joints are not inert hinges; they are living structures that depend on movement for nourishment, lubrication, and sensory feedback.

Modern physiology echoes this insight. Synovial fluid circulation, cartilage nutrition, and neuromuscular coordination all improve with **gentle, continuous motion**. What matters is not force, but consistency and quality of movement.

Tai Chi treats joints as participants in an integrated system rather than isolated mechanical components. Movements are circular rather than linear, transitions are gradual, and range of motion is explored without pushing into pain. This approach supports circulation while minimizing inflammatory stress.

In Tai Chi, joints are not challenged aggressively; they are **invited to participate**.

Tai Chi's Non-Compressional Strength

A key therapeutic advantage of Tai Chi in arthritis and rheumatism lies in how it develops strength. Rather than emphasizing maximal contraction or repetitive loading, Tai Chi cultivates **structural alignment and coordinated support**.

Strength emerges from:
- Balanced weight distribution
- Efficient use of gravity
- Coordinated engagement of multiple muscle groups
- Reduced reliance on isolated joints

This non-compressional strengthening protects vulnerable joints while enhancing overall stability. The body learns to support itself through organization rather than force. Over time, this reduces compensatory tension and uneven loading—common contributors to chronic pain.

Because Tai Chi movements are slow and controlled, participants can remain within pain-free or low-pain ranges, reinforcing the association between movement and safety rather than threat.

Pain Reduction Through Movement Confidence

Chronic pain is not solely a product of tissue damage. It is shaped by fear, anticipation, and learned avoidance. When movement is consistently associated with pain, the nervous system becomes hypervigilant, amplifying discomfort and restricting motion further.

Tai Chi interrupts this cycle by creating repeated experiences of **successful, non-threatening movement**. Participants learn that they can move without triggering flare-ups, that joints can remain stable during transitions, and that discomfort does not inevitably escalate into injury.

This restoration of confidence is therapeutically significant. As fear decreases, movement becomes smoother. As movement becomes smoother, stress on joints decreases. Pain, in turn, often diminishes—not because it is suppressed, but because the conditions that sustain it are gradually altered.

Research Findings in Arthritis and Rheumatic Conditions

Clinical studies examining Tai Chi in osteoarthritis, rheumatoid arthritis, and related conditions have reported:

- Reduced joint pain
- Improved physical function
- Increased range of motion
- Improved balance and stability
- Enhanced mood and reduced stress

- Better adherence compared to conventional exercise programs

While outcomes vary by condition and study design, the overall pattern is consistent: Tai Chi is safe, well-tolerated, and associated with functional improvements that matter to daily life.

Notably, participants often continue Tai Chi practice beyond study periods, suggesting that its benefits are not only measurable, but **experientially meaningful**.

Program Design for Arthritic Populations

Therapeutic Tai Chi for arthritis and rheumatism requires careful attention to adaptation. The goal is not technical mastery, but sustainable engagement.

Key principles include:
- Avoiding end-range loading
- Respecting pain signals without reinforcing fear
- Emphasizing smooth transitions over large ranges
- Allowing seated practice when needed
- Encouraging self-pacing and rest

Instructors must resist the temptation to "push progress." In arthritic populations, progress often appears as **greater ease**, not increased range or speed. Success is measured in reduced stiffness, improved daily function, and renewed willingness to move.

Reframing Arthritis Care

Tai Chi invites a reframing of arthritis care away from battle metaphors and toward **collaboration with the body**. Rather than fighting pain or forcing joints to perform, practitioners learn to listen, adjust, and adapt.

This reframing has ethical as well as therapeutic implications. It respects the lived experience of chronic illness and restores agency to individuals who are often defined by limitation.

Tai Chi does not promise cure. It offers something more realistic and, in many cases, more valuable: a way to move **without aggression**, preserving function, dignity, and quality of life over time.

Chapter Summary

Arthritis and rheumatic conditions challenge conventional exercise approaches that rely on force and repetition. Tai Chi offers a gentle, integrative alternative that supports joint circulation, non-compressional strength, and movement confidence. By emphasizing smooth transitions, alignment, and adaptability, Tai Chi reduces pain, improves function, and encourages sustained participation. Its therapeutic value lies not in overcoming limitation, but in working intelligently within it.

PART III:
INTEGRATION INTO CARE SETTINGS

PART III:
INTRODUCTION INTO
CANCER CELLS

Chapter Six

Respiratory Regulation, Sleep, and Apnea

Breath as a Regulatory System

Breathing is often treated as a mechanical function: air moves in, air moves out. Clinically, however, breath is one of the body's most sensitive indicators of overall regulation. It reflects neurological state, emotional tone, postural organization, and autonomic balance simultaneously.

Disordered breathing rarely exists in isolation. Shallow respiration, breath holding, irregular rhythm, and poor coordination between breath and movement are commonly associated with chronic stress, neurological disease, musculoskeletal restriction, and sleep disturbance. Over time, these patterns reinforce fatigue, anxiety, pain sensitivity, and impaired recovery.

From both Chinese Medicine and modern physiology, breath is understood not simply as oxygen exchange, but as a **regulatory interface**—*a point at which voluntary and involuntary systems meet. Tai Chi engages this interface directly.*

Sympathetic and Parasympathetic Balance

Many respiratory and sleep-related disorders reflect an imbalance in the autonomic nervous system. Excessive sympathetic activation—associated with vigilance, stress, and arousal—disrupts respiratory rhythm and interferes with restorative sleep. Even at rest, individuals may remain in a state of physiological readiness that prevents true recovery.

Sleep apnea, fragmented sleep, and chronic insomnia often coexist with heightened autonomic arousal. While mechanical factors such as airway obstruction play a role in apnea, regulation of muscle tone, breath timing, and nervous system activation also contributes significantly.

Tai Chi supports parasympathetic engagement not through forced relaxation, but through **coordinated, rhythmic movement paired with calm attention**. This combination gently downregulates arousal without suppressing alertness.

Tai Chi and Diaphragmatic Coordination

One of the most consistent physiological effects of Tai Chi practice is improved diaphragmatic breathing. This improvement does not arise from explicit breath control exercises alone, but from changes in posture, timing, and muscular coordination.

Tai Chi encourages:

- Upright, relaxed spinal alignment
- Reduced accessory muscle overuse
- Coordinated movement of trunk and limbs
- Natural synchronization of breath with motion

As postural tension decreases, the diaphragm regains mobility. Breathing becomes deeper, slower, and more efficient—not through effort, but through *removal of interference*. This shift supports improved oxygen exchange and reduces respiratory fatigue.

For individuals with chronic respiratory limitation, this can translate into greater ease of breathing during daily activities and reduced sensation of breathlessness.

Sleep Quality and Autonomic Downregulation

Sleep quality depends not only on duration, but on the nervous system's ability to transition into restorative states. Many individuals with chronic illness report spending adequate time in bed while waking unrefreshed. This reflects incomplete downregulation rather than simple sleep deprivation.

Tai Chi appears to support sleep through multiple pathways:
- Reduction of baseline physiological arousal
- Improved respiratory rhythm
- Decreased musculoskeletal tension
- Enhanced body awareness
- Improved emotional regulation

Because Tai Chi practice is neither exhausting nor stimulating, it can be integrated safely into daily routines, including earlier evening hours, without disrupting sleep onset. Over time, regular practice helps retrain the nervous system to recognize and inhabit calmer states more reliably.

Tai Chi and Sleep Apnea: A Supportive Role

Tai Chi is not a primary treatment for sleep apnea and should not be presented as a substitute for medical management. However, it may play a supportive role in addressing contributing factors that exacerbate apnea and related sleep disturbances.

These include:
- Poor postural alignment affecting airway mechanics

- Reduced respiratory muscle coordination
- Chronic sympathetic dominance
- Fragmented sleep architecture

By improving posture, breath coordination, and autonomic balance, Tai Chi may complement conventional treatments such as CPAP or oral appliances. Some individuals report improved tolerance of these devices when overall respiratory comfort improves.

The therapeutic value of Tai Chi in this context lies not in mechanical correction, but in **system-wide regulation**.

Adaptations for Limited Mobility and Fatigue

Respiratory and sleep disorders often coexist with fatigue, neurological impairment, or reduced mobility. Tai Chi's adaptability is therefore critical.

Seated Tai Chi emphasizes:

- Trunk expansion and release
- Coordinated arm movement
- Gentle rotational patterns
- Breath–movement synchronization

Standing practice, when appropriate, adds:

- Postural alignment
- Weight distribution
- Increased respiratory demand within safe limits

Sessions can be brief, interspersed with rest, and adjusted dynamically based on daily capacity. Therapeutic Tai Chi respects variability rather than resisting it.

Restoring the Experience of Ease

Perhaps the most important contribution Tai Chi offers individuals with respiratory and sleep disturbances is experiential rather than technical. Many people living with chronic breath or sleep issues develop a persistent sense of effort—breathing feels labored, rest feels elusive, and the body never fully settles.

Tai Chi reintroduces the experience of *ease*. Through slow, coordinated movement, participants rediscover breathing that supports rather than resists activity. This experiential shift often carries into daily life and nighttime rest.

Ease is not a luxury in chronic illness; it is a therapeutic necessity.

Chapter Summary

Respiratory and sleep disturbances reflect broader failures of autonomic and postural regulation rather than isolated mechanical defects. Tai Chi supports respiratory efficiency, diaphragmatic coordination, and parasympathetic engagement through slow, integrated movement and attentive practice. While not a substitute for medical treatment, Tai Chi offers a safe, adaptable method for improving breath regulation, sleep quality, and overall recovery—particularly in individuals with chronic illness or fatigue.

Chapter Seven

Tai Chi in Clinical and Residential Environments

Why Care Settings Need More Than Activities

In clinical and residential environments—assisted living, memory care, rehabilitation centers, and long-term care facilities—movement is often treated as an "activity." Activities fill time, provide stimulation, and offer social engagement. While valuable, this framing is insufficient for populations living with chronic illness, neurological impairment, or functional decline.

What these settings require are not merely activities, but **therapeutic structures**—interventions that support stability, autonomy, and regulation while respecting medical complexity and vulnerability.

Tai Chi meets this need precisely because it does not demand performance, competition, or exertion. It functions as **therapeutic movement**, capable of adapting to fluctuating capacity while delivering measurable functional benefits.

Assisted Living and Memory Care

Assisted living and memory care populations face overlapping challenges: fall risk, cognitive impairment, anxiety, reduced mobility, and loss of routine. Traditional exercise programs often fail in these environments because they rely on instruction, repetition, and motivation—capacities that may be compromised.

Tai Chi addresses these challenges through:

- Predictable, repetitive movement patterns
- Slow pace that reduces cognitive load
- Visual mirroring rather than verbal instruction
- Emphasis on rhythm and continuity
- Seated and supported options for safety

In memory care settings, Tai Chi's value extends beyond physical outcomes. The practice promotes calm engagement, reduces agitation, and provides a structured sensory experience that does not rely on short-term memory. Participants can join and rejoin the movement flow without feeling lost or corrected.

Tai Chi becomes less an "exercise class" and more a **regulatory environment**—one that supports both body and mind.

Rehabilitation and Neurological Clinics

In rehabilitation settings, Tai Chi complements rather than replaces physical and occupational therapy. Its strength lies in addressing aspects of movement often underemphasized in conventional rehab: continuity, timing, internal coordination, and confidence.

Patients recovering from stroke, living with Parkinson's disease, or managing chronic neurological conditions often demonstrate adequate strength but impaired integration. Tai Chi offers a bridge between structured therapy sessions and independent movement by reinforcing:

- Postural control
- Weight shifting

- Gait preparation
- Attention–movement coupling

Because Tai Chi is low impact and adaptable, it can be introduced early in rehabilitation and maintained long after discharge. This continuity supports long-term functional gains that episodic therapy alone may not sustain.

Community and Preventive Health Programs

Community-based Tai Chi programs play a critical role in preventive health, particularly among older adults. By addressing balance, coordination, and confidence before severe decline occurs, Tai Chi reduces downstream healthcare utilization.

From a public health perspective, Tai Chi offers:

- Broad accessibility
- Low infrastructure requirements
- Minimal risk
- High participant retention
- Scalability across diverse populations

Programs delivered through community centers, senior centers, and faith-based organizations often reach individuals who would not otherwise engage in preventive care. Tai Chi thus functions as both a therapeutic and a **community health intervention**.

Safety, Liability, and Scope of Practice

For institutions, safety and liability are paramount. Tai Chi's suitability in care settings depends on clear boundaries and professional standards.

Key considerations include:

- Instructor training in therapeutic adaptation

- Clear screening and contraindication awareness
- Emphasis on participant choice and self-pacing
- Avoidance of medical claims or diagnosis
- Coordination with clinical staff when appropriate

Therapeutic Tai Chi instructors do not replace healthcare providers. They operate within a defined scope: facilitating safe movement experiences that support function and regulation. When properly implemented, Tai Chi programs carry low injury risk and high tolerance across populations.

Collaboration with Medical and Care Staff

Successful integration of Tai Chi into care environments depends on collaboration rather than isolation. Instructors must communicate clearly with nurses, therapists, and administrators, aligning goals and expectations.

Effective collaboration includes:

- Understanding facility protocols
- Adapting sessions to daily clinical rhythms
- Sharing observational feedback (without diagnosis)
- Respecting medical limitations and precautions

When Tai Chi is understood as part of a broader care ecosystem, its benefits are amplified. Staff often report improved resident engagement, calmer group dynamics, and reduced resistance to movement activities.

From Program to Culture

The most effective Tai Chi programs do more than deliver sessions; they influence institutional culture. Over time, Tai Chi can reshape how movement is perceived—from a task imposed on residents to an experience shared with them.

When movement becomes predictable, safe, and dignified, participation increases. When participants feel respected rather than corrected, engagement deepens. Tai Chi models a way of working with vulnerable populations that emphasizes **presence over performance**.

This cultural shift has implications beyond Tai Chi itself. It fosters environments where regulation, patience, and attentiveness become normative values—qualities essential to humane care.

Chapter Summary

Clinical and residential environments require therapeutic movement approaches that prioritize safety, adaptability, and regulation. Tai Chi integrates effectively into assisted living, memory care, rehabilitation, and community health settings by supporting balance, coordination, and calm engagement without imposing excessive cognitive or physical demands. When implemented collaboratively and ethically, Tai Chi functions not merely as an activity, but as a therapeutic structure that enhances care culture and quality of life.

Chapter Eight

Designing Therapeutic Tai Chi Programs

Why Therapeutic Tai Chi Is Not Generic Tai Chi

Not all Tai Chi is therapeutic, and not all Tai Chi instructors are prepared to work in clinical or vulnerable populations. Traditional Tai Chi training often emphasizes form precision, lineage, performance, or martial application. While valuable in their own contexts, these priorities do not translate automatically into therapeutic environments.

Therapeutic Tai Chi begins from a different premise: **the participant's regulatory capacity, not the form, is primary**. Movements are selected, adapted, and sequenced based on function, safety, and adaptability rather than aesthetic or traditional completeness.

This distinction must be made explicit. Without it, Tai Chi risks being misapplied, misunderstood, or dismissed within healthcare settings.

Instructor Training Requirements

Therapeutic Tai Chi instructors require training beyond technical proficiency. They must understand how movement interacts with chronic illness, neurological impairment, pain, fatigue, and cognitive limitation.

Core competencies include:

- Functional anatomy and basic neurophysiology
- Principles of balance and fall prevention
- Adaptation for seated and supported practice
- Recognition of fatigue, pain escalation, and distress
- Clear communication without medical diagnosis
- Trauma-informed and dignity-preserving instruction

Equally important is **what instructors must not do**: diagnose conditions, offer medical advice, or promise outcomes. Therapeutic Tai Chi operates alongside healthcare, not in place of it.

Assessment and Functional Orientation

Therapeutic Tai Chi does not rely on formal medical assessment. However, it does require **functional observation**.

Instructors should attend to:

- Postural organization
- Weight-bearing capacity
- Movement initiation and hesitation
- Range of motion within comfort
- Attention and engagement
- Emotional response to movement

These observations guide adaptation. Progress is measured not by mastery of forms, but by increased ease, stability, and participation. Improvement may appear as reduced fear, smoother transitions, or willingness to move rather than expanded range or endurance.

Adaptation and Progression Principles

Progression in therapeutic Tai Chi is non-linear. Capacity fluctuates, particularly in chronic illness and neurodegenerative conditions. Programs must be designed to accommodate variability without framing it as regression.

Key principles include:

- Begin within the participant's comfort zone
- Favor repetition over novelty
- Maintain predictable structure
- Introduce complexity gradually
- Allow frequent rest without stigma
- Normalize modification as success

Seated practice is not a preliminary stage to be "outgrown." For many participants, it remains the most effective and dignified form of engagement. Standing and walking elements are introduced only when they enhance safety and confidence.

Ethical Boundaries and Language

Language shapes experience. In therapeutic contexts, instructors must avoid metaphors or promises that create unrealistic expectations or dependency.

Ethical practice includes:

- Avoiding claims of cure
- Framing Tai Chi as supportive, not corrective
- Emphasizing participant choice
- Respecting pain signals
- Avoiding competition or comparison

Tai Chi becomes therapeutic not because it is gentle, but because it is **respectful**—of limits, autonomy, and lived experience.

Measuring Outcomes Without Medicalizing the Practice

Institutions often require evidence of effectiveness. Therapeutic Tai Chi can provide measurable outcomes without becoming medicalized.

Appropriate indicators include:
- Reduced fall incidence
- Improved balance confidence
- Increased participation
- Improved functional mobility
- Enhanced calm engagement
- Improved quality-of-life measures

Subjective experience matters. Participant reports of ease, confidence, and well-being are not secondary outcomes; they are central to therapeutic value.

Program Structure and Sustainability

Effective programs are simple, consistent, and sustainable. Overly complex curricula increase instructor burden and reduce accessibility.

Sustainable programs typically feature:
- Regular, predictable scheduling
- Small to moderate group sizes
- Clear session structure
- Ongoing instructor support
- Integration into existing care routines

When Tai Chi is treated as an add-on, it remains fragile. When it is integrated into institutional rhythms, it becomes resilient.

Professionalizing Therapeutic Tai Chi

For Tai Chi to function as a credible therapeutic modality, it must be

professionalized without being medicalized. This includes:
- Clear training pathways
- Ethical standards
- Scope-of-practice clarity
- Collaboration with healthcare professionals
- Ongoing education and reflection

Professionalization protects participants, instructors, and institutions alike. It ensures that Tai Chi's growing presence in healthcare is grounded in responsibility rather than enthusiasm alone.

Chapter Summary

Therapeutic Tai Chi is a distinct practice requiring specialized training, ethical clarity, and functional orientation. Its effectiveness depends not on technical mastery, but on adaptability, observation, and respect for participant capacity. When designed thoughtfully, therapeutic Tai Chi programs are safe, sustainable, and institutionally credible—supporting regulation, dignity, and long-term engagement without overstepping medical boundaries.

PART IV: THE FUTURE OF THERAPEUTIC TAI CHI

Chapter Nine

From Complementary to Essential

The Shift Toward Non-Pharmacological Care

Healthcare systems around the world are undergoing a quiet but profound shift. While pharmacological and surgical interventions remain indispensable, there is growing recognition that many of the most burdensome conditions of modern societies cannot be solved through medication alone. Chronic illness, neurodegeneration, frailty, and age-related decline demand approaches that support **ongoing regulation rather than episodic intervention**.

This shift is not ideological. It is driven by necessity.

Rising healthcare costs, aging populations, workforce shortages, and the cumulative effects of long-term medication use have forced systems to reconsider how care is delivered. Increasingly, attention has turned to non-pharmacological interventions that improve function, reduce risk, and support independence without adding complexity or harm.

Tai Chi fits squarely within this emerging paradigm.

Cost, Prevention, and Functional Independence

From a systems perspective, small functional improvements can yield disproportionate benefits. Preventing a fall, delaying institutionalization, or preserving mobility for an additional year can significantly reduce healthcare utilization and associated costs.

Tai Chi contributes to these outcomes by:
- Reducing fall risk
- Supporting balance and gait stability
- Encouraging regular movement
- Improving confidence and engagement
- Enhancing adherence through positive experience

Unlike many preventive interventions, Tai Chi does not require expensive equipment, specialized facilities, or ongoing consumables. Its cost structure is modest, and its scalability high. This makes it particularly attractive for public health initiatives and community-based programs.

Importantly, Tai Chi's benefits accrue over time. It is not a quick fix, but a **maintenance strategy**—precisely what chronic care requires.

Aging Societies and the Question of Dignity

As populations age, the question is no longer whether people will live longer, but **how they will live longer**. Functional decline, loss of autonomy, and social isolation are among the greatest threats to well-being in later life.

Tai Chi addresses these challenges in ways that extend beyond physical metrics. It offers older adults a way to remain engaged, capable, and embodied. Movement is not framed as a test to be passed, but as a shared experience that adapts to changing capacity.

This emphasis on dignity matters. When care prioritizes function without humiliation and safety without infantilization, participation increases and outcomes improve. Tai Chi models this balance.

Why Tai Chi Aligns With Public Health Strategy

Public health interventions succeed when they are accessible, acceptable, and sustainable. Tai Chi meets these criteria across diverse populations.

Its alignment with public health goals includes:
- Broad applicability across age groups and conditions
- Minimal contraindications
- Cultural adaptability
- Compatibility with existing healthcare infrastructure
- Capacity to be delivered in group settings

Moreover, Tai Chi promotes self-efficacy. Participants are not passive recipients of care; they are active contributors to their own regulation. This aligns with contemporary public health emphasis on empowerment and prevention.

Complementary or Essential?

The label "complementary" has often relegated practices like Tai Chi to the periphery of healthcare—useful, perhaps, but optional. Yet as healthcare challenges evolve, this distinction becomes less meaningful.

When an intervention:
- Improves function
- Reduces risk
- Enhances quality of life
- Carries low risk
- Encourages sustained engagement

—it begins to resemble an **essential component of care**, particularly for populations living with chronic conditions.

Tai Chi does not compete with medicine. It complements it in the truest sense: by addressing dimensions of health that medicine alone cannot fully reach. In doing so, it becomes indispensable.

Integrating Tai Chi Into Care Pathways

For Tai Chi to transition from complementary to essential, integration must be intentional. This includes:

- Recognition within care planning
- Collaboration with clinical teams
- Inclusion in preventive health strategies
- Support for instructor training and standards
- Ongoing evaluation and refinement

Integration does not mean medicalization. Tai Chi retains its distinct character precisely because it operates through experience rather than intervention. Its value lies in **how it works**, not in how it is classified.

A Model for Future Therapeutic Practices

Tai Chi offers more than a single modality; it provides a model for how therapeutic practices can evolve. It demonstrates that:

- Regulation can be trained
- Movement can be medicine without being aggressive
- Care can be effective without being invasive
- Tradition and science can coexist without dilution

As healthcare continues to confront complex, chronic challenges, such models will become increasingly important.

Chapter Summary

As healthcare systems shift toward managing chronic illness, aging, and functional decline, non-pharmacological interventions that support regulation and independence become increasingly essential. Tai Chi aligns with this shift by offering a low-risk, scalable approach that improves balance, confidence, and quality of life. Its growing integration into care pathways reflects not a trend, but a structural response to the realities of modern healthcare.

Chapter Ten

Tai Chi as a Medical Culture, Not a Technique

Why Tai Chi Resists Standardization

Modern healthcare is built on standardization. Protocols, guidelines, and reproducible interventions are essential for safety and scalability. Yet not all therapeutic value can be fully captured in standardized procedures. Tai Chi resists standardization not because it lacks rigor, but because its effectiveness depends on **responsiveness rather than prescription**.

Tai Chi does not operate through fixed doses or uniform execution. It works through continuous adjustment—of posture, timing, attention, and effort—within the lived reality of each participant. This adaptability is not a weakness; it is the source of Tai Chi's therapeutic power.

Attempts to reduce Tai Chi to a sequence of techniques risk stripping it of precisely what makes it effective: its capacity to meet variability without forcing conformity.

Why That Resistance Is a Strength

In chronic illness, neurodegeneration, and aging, variability is the rule rather than the exception. Capacity fluctuates. Symptoms change. Good days and difficult days coexist. Therapies that demand consistency from the patient often fail when consistency is no longer possible.

Tai Chi accommodates variability by design. Movements can be scaled, slowed, simplified, or supported without loss of meaning. Participation does not depend on performance, memory, or endurance. It depends on **presence.**

This quality allows Tai Chi to remain effective across stages of illness and across diverse care settings. Its flexibility is not an accommodation; it is an intrinsic feature.

The Ethics of Teaching Therapeutic Tai Chi

Teaching Tai Chi in therapeutic contexts carries ethical responsibilities. Instructors work with individuals who may be vulnerable—physically, cognitively, or emotionally. The goal is not to improve performance, but to **support dignity, agency, and safety.**

Ethical teaching requires:

- Respect for limits without reinforcing helplessness
- Clear boundaries around medical claims
- Attentiveness to signs of distress or fatigue
- Willingness to adapt without judgment
- Commitment to ongoing learning and humility

In this sense, therapeutic Tai Chi is as much about *how* one teaches as *what* one teaches. Technique matters, but attitude matters more.

Tai Chi as Ongoing Regulation, Not Treatment

Western medicine often frames care as a sequence of treatments aimed at resolution. Tai Chi proposes a different model: **ongoing regulation.** Regulation is not something achieved once and then maintained automatically. It is a dynamic process that requires continuous participation. Tai Chi trains this participation. It teaches individuals how to notice imbalance early, respond gently, and reestablish coherence.

This model aligns with the realities of chronic conditions, where cure may not be possible, but quality of life remains deeply influenced by how one lives within limitation.

Responsibility Reclaimed Through Movement

Chronic illness often erodes a person's sense of responsibility—not in the moral sense, but in the experiential one. Decisions about the body are transferred to clinicians, medications, and institutions. While necessary, this transfer can leave individuals feeling passive and disconnected.

Tai Chi reintroduces responsibility in a humane way. It does not ask participants to control outcomes they cannot control. It asks them to **participate in regulation where participation remains possible**.

Through movement, responsibility becomes embodied rather than abstract. It is felt in posture, breath, and balance. This reclamation of agency has therapeutic value independent of measurable outcomes.

A Culture of Care, Not a Collection of Techniques

Ultimately, Tai Chi offers more than a set of movements. It offers a **culture of care**—one that values attentiveness over force, adaptation over correction, and continuity over intensity.

When integrated into healthcare environments, Tai Chi models a different relationship to the body: one that is neither adversarial nor dismissive, but collaborative. This cultural dimension explains why Tai Chi's impact often extends beyond individual sessions, influencing how participants and caregivers alike think about movement, aging, and illness.

The Future of Therapeutic Movement

As healthcare continues to evolve, the need for practices that support regulation, dignity, and long-term engagement will only grow. Tai Chi stands as an example of how ancient practices can inform modern care—not by resisting science, but by addressing dimensions of human experience that science alone cannot fully capture.

Its future lies not in replacing medicine, but in **humanizing it**.

Book Conclusion

This book has argued that Tai Chi is best understood not as an alternative therapy, but as an embodied extension of Chinese Medicine's regulatory logic—one that modern healthcare has increasingly recognized as essential.

Across balance, neurological disease, chronic pain, respiratory regulation, and institutional care, Tai Chi offers a coherent, adaptable, and humane approach to therapeutic movement.

Its value lies not in curing disease, but in restoring conditions under which life can be lived with greater stability, confidence, and dignity.

Postscript

Tai Chi Health & Wellness USA (TCHWUSA)

This book has argued that Tai Chi is best understood not as an alternative technique, but as an embodied form of regulation—one that modern healthcare increasingly requires as it confronts chronic illness, aging, and functional decline.

The ideas developed here are not theoretical alone. They inform the ongoing work of *Tai Chi Health & Wellness USA (TCHWUSA)*, an organization founded by Maurice (Moshe) Pitchon dedicated to integrating **therapeutic Tai Chi** into clinical, residential, and community health settings.

TCHWUSA was created to address a practical gap: while research increasingly supports Tai Chi's therapeutic value, healthcare environments require **standards, training, ethical clarity, and institutional coordination** in order to implement it responsibly. TCHWUSA operates as an umbrella organization bringing these elements together.

Two Complementary Platforms

TCHWUSA functions through two interconnected platforms, each serving a distinct but related role:

- https://taichihealthwellnessusa.net/
- This platform focuses on *therapeutic Tai Chi programs* for health, aging, and chronic disease management. It supports

program design and delivery in assisted living communities, rehabilitation centers, memory care settings, and community health initiatives. The emphasis is on safety, adaptability, and dignity in movement for vulnerable populations.
- https://www.tchwusa.com/
- This platform is dedicated to *professional training, instructor certification, and organizational collaboration.* It establishes standards for therapeutic Tai Chi instruction, supports a national and international professional network, and serves as a hub for educators, instructors, and institutions committed to evidence-based practice.

Together, these platforms reflect a central principle of this book: therapeutic Tai Chi must be supported both *in practice* and **in** *professional culture.*

Advancing the Field: International Symposium

In addition to its ongoing programs and training initiatives, TCHWU-SA is the organizer of the:

TCHWUSA International Symposium on Tai Chi for
Wellness and Chronic Disease Management
June 15–17, 2027 | South Florida

The symposium is conceived as a non-competitive, professional forum bringing together healthcare professionals, researchers, instructors, administrators, and organizations engaged in the therapeutic application of Tai Chi. Its purpose is not advocacy, but **exchange**—advancing clinical understanding, ethical practice, and institutional integration of Tai Chi in health and aging contexts.

A Living Framework

The work of TCHWUSA is not presented here as a conclusion, but as a continuation. As healthcare systems evolve, so too must the ways in which therapeutic movement is understood, taught, and applied. The platforms described above are intended to remain responsive to emerging research, clinical realities, and ethical responsibilities.

If this book has argued that Tai Chi is a medical culture rather than a technique, TCHWUSA represents one attempt to give that culture **organizational form**—so that the principles of regulation, responsibility, and dignity explored in these pages can be lived out in real care environments.

APPENDICES

APPENDICES

Appendix A

Program Safety Checklist

Therapeutic Tai Chi programs must prioritize safety, dignity, and adaptability, particularly when delivered to older adults or individuals with chronic illness or neurological impairment.

The following principles define minimum safety standards for program implementation:

- Participation is always voluntary; rest and modification are normalized
- Movements remain slow, controlled, and reversible
- No forced range of motion or end-range loading
- No ballistic, rapid, or impact-based movements
- Pain is treated as information, not resistance
- Seated practice is considered a complete and valid format
- Environmental hazards (flooring, spacing, lighting) are addressed in advance
- Instructors remain attentive to fatigue, dizziness, confusion, or distress

Therapeutic Tai Chi instructors do not diagnose medical conditions, adjust medications, or offer prognostic claims. Programs should be coordinated, when appropriate, with facility staff and operate within clearly defined scope-of-practice boundaries.

Appendix B

Instructor Competency Framework

Effective therapeutic Tai Chi instruction depends less on technical form mastery than on professional judgment, adaptability, and ethical clarity.

Minimum competencies include:

- Understanding of basic functional anatomy and balance principles
- Ability to adapt movements for seated, supported, and standing participants
- Awareness of fall risk and neurological vulnerability
- Clear, calm, non-directive communication
- Sensitivity to cognitive, emotional, and cultural differences
- Commitment to participant dignity and autonomy

Instructors must also demonstrate clear boundaries, including:

- Avoiding medical diagnosis or treatment claims
- Refraining from promises of cure or disease modification
- Respecting institutional policies and clinical authority
- Maintaining professional conduct in all care settings

This framework is intended to support professionalization without medicalization, ensuring that therapeutic Tai Chi remains safe, credible, and ethically grounded as it continues to expand into healthcare environments.

Appendix R

Instructor Competency Framework

Appendix C

Chinese medicine term	Functional / clinical interpretation
Qi	Coordinated physiological function
Yin–yang	Dynamic balance between opposing processes
Rooting	Efficient ground reaction & postural stability
Shen	Attention, presence, cognitive-emotional regulation
Stagnation	Impaired circulation or coordination
Balance	Neurological integration, not static posture

Appendix C

Appendix D

Modern Wellness Tai Chi Sequence Vocabulary

This system keeps the mind-body-spirit feel but rebrands it into language that feels natural in a modern western facility, fitness studio, wellness retreat, or even an app for beginners.

Opening & Foundations

- Commencement → **Grounded Breath**
- Parting the Wild Horse's Mane → **Flow Reach**
- White Crane Spreads Wings → **Open Stretch**

Core Balancing Moves

- Grasp the Bird's Tail → **Core Flow**
- Brush Knee and Twist Step → **Balance Sweep**
- Play the Lute → **Center Pause**
- Repulse Monkey → **Step Back Flow**

Rotational & Rooted Strength

- Wave Hands Like Clouds → **Cloud Flow**

- Single Whip → **Power Arc**
- Fair Lady Works Shuttles → **Cross Reach**
- Needle at Sea Bottom → **Ground Point**
- Fan Through the Back → **Energy Fan**

Stamina & Directional Flow

- Kick with Heel → **Power Kick**
- Snake Creeps Down → **Low Flow**
- Golden Rooster Stands on One Leg → **Balance Stand**
- Step Up, Deflect, Parry and Punch → **Power Strike**

Closing & Integration

- Apparent Close-Up → **Energy Seal**
- Cross Hands → **Center Wrap**
- Closing Form → **Return to Breath**

Bibliography

The therapeutic claims discussed in this book draw on a broad and heterogeneous body of research examining Tai Chi across clinical, community, and institutional settings. Rather than relying on a single methodological approach, the literature reflects the complexity of Tai Chi as a multicomponent intervention.

Most studies referenced fall into one or more of the following categories:

- Randomized controlled trials comparing Tai Chi to usual care, resistance training, or stretching
- Longitudinal observational studies in aging or neurologically impaired populations
- Systematic reviews and meta-analyses focused on balance, mobility, pain, and quality of life
- Pragmatic studies conducted in community, assisted living, or rehabilitation settings

It is important to note that Tai Chi does not lend itself easily to reductionist research designs. Its effects emerge from the interaction of posture, movement, attention, breath, and social context. For this reason, outcome-based research—falls, balance confidence, functional mobility, adherence, and participant experience—has proven more informative than attempts to isolate single variables.

This book uses research selectively and structurally: not to exhaustively catalog studies, but to justify the therapeutic organization of chapters around functional capacities rather than disease labels. Readers seeking detailed statistical analysis are encouraged to consult the original sources listed in this bibliography.

Foundational & Theoretical Works

Kaptchuk, Ted J. *The Web That Has No Weaver: Understanding Chinese Medicine*. 2nd ed. New York: McGraw-Hill, 2000.

Unschuld, Paul U. *Medicine in China: A History of Ideas*. 25th Anniversary ed. Berkeley: University of California Press, 2010.

Wayne, Peter M., and Ted J. Kaptchuk. "Challenges Inherent to Tai Chi Research: Part I—Tai Chi as a Complex Multicomponent Intervention." *Journal of Alternative and Complementary Medicine* 14, no. 1 (2008): 95–102.

Wayne, Peter M. *The Harvard Medical School Guide to Tai Chi*. Boston: Shambhala, 2013.

Langevin, Helene M., and Peter M. Wayne. "What Is the Point? The Problem with Acupuncture Research That No One Wants to Talk About." *Journal of Alternative and Complementary Medicine* 24, no. 3 (2018): 200–207.

Balance, Fall Prevention, and Aging (Chapter Three)

Li, Fangyu, Peter Harmer, Karen Fitzgerald, et al. "Tai Chi and Postural Stability in Patients with Parkinson's Disease." *New England Journal of Medicine* 366, no. 6 (2012): 511–519.

Wolf, Steven L., Hilary X. Barnhart, Nancy G. Kutner, Elizabeth McNeely, Cindy Coogler, and Ti Xu. "Reducing Frailty and Falls in Older Persons: An Investigation of Tai Chi and Computerized Balance Training." *Journal of the American Geriatrics Society* 44, no. 5 (1996): 489–497.

Gillespie, Lesley D., M. Clare Robertson, William J. Gillespie, et al. "Interventions for Preventing Falls in Older People Living in the Community." *Cochrane Database of Systematic Reviews* (2012):

CD007146.

Sherrington, Catherine, Nicola J. Fairhall, Georgia K. Wallbank, et al. "Exercise for Preventing Falls in Older People Living in the Community." *British Journal of Sports Medicine* 54, no. 15 (2020): 905–911.

Parkinson's Disease and Neurological Conditions (Chapter Four)

Hackney, Madeleine E., and Gammon M. Earhart. "Tai Chi Improves Balance and Mobility in People with Parkinson Disease." *Gait & Posture* 28, no. 3 (2008): 456–460.

Li, Fangyu, Peter Harmer, Yijie Liu, et al. "A Randomized Controlled Trial of Tai Chi for Parkinson's Disease." *Movement Disorders* 29, no. 9 (2014): 1200–1207.

Klein, Penelope J., Linda Rivers, et al. "Tai Chi for Balance, Mobility, and Gait in Parkinson Disease." *Parkinson's Disease* (2014): Article ID 318468.

Mak, Maggie M. K. Y., Irene S. K. Wong-Yu, Xia Shen, and Cecilia L. Chung. "Long-Term Effects of Exercise and Physical Therapy in People with Parkinson Disease." *Nature Reviews Neurology* 13, no. 11 (2017): 689–703.

Arthritis, Rheumatism, and Chronic Pain (Chapter Five)

Wang, Chenchen, Charles H. Schmid, Robert Rones, et al. "A Randomized Trial of Tai Chi for Fibromyalgia." *New England Journal of Medicine* 363, no. 8 (2010): 743–754.

Wang, Chenchen, Charles H. Schmid, Patricia L. Hibberd, et al. "Tai Chi Is Effective in Treating Knee Osteoarthritis: A Randomized

Controlled Trial." *Arthritis & Rheumatism* 61, no. 11 (2009): 1545–1553.

Lee, Myeong Soo, Max H. Pittler, and Edzard Ernst. "Tai Chi for Rheumatoid Arthritis: A Systematic Review." *Rheumatology* 47, no. 12 (2008): 1747–1751.

Song, Ryu, Bonnie L. Roberts, Eun Ok Lee, Paul Lam, and Sung Il Bae. "A Randomized Study of the Effects of Tai Chi on Muscle Strength, Bone Mineral Density, and Fear of Falling in Women with Osteoarthritis." *Journal of Rheumatology* 37, no. 7 (2010): 1556–1563.

Respiration, Sleep, and Autonomic Regulation (Chapter Six)

Irwin, Michael R., Rebecca Olmstead, and Salma J. Motivala. "Improving Sleep Quality in Older Adults with Moderate Sleep Complaints: A Randomized Controlled Trial of Tai Chi Chih." *Sleep* 31, no. 7 (2008): 1001–1008.

Yeh, Gloria Y., Chenchen Wang, Peter M. Wayne, and Russell Phillips. "Tai Chi Exercise for Patients with Cardiovascular Conditions and Risk Factors: A Systematic Review." *Journal of Cardiopulmonary Rehabilitation and Prevention* 29, no. 3 (2009): 152–160.

Lan, Chien-Yu, Shao-Yu Chen, and Jau-Sheng Lai. "Relative Exercise Intensity of Tai Chi Chuan Is Similar in Different Ages and Genders." *American Journal of Chinese Medicine* 32, no. 1 (2004): 151–160.

Wayne, Peter M., Brad Manor, Vera Novak, et al. "A Systems Biology Approach to Tai Chi Research." *Journal of Alternative and Complementary Medicine* 19, no. 8 (2013): 1–8.

Institutional, Community, and Public Health

Applications (Chapters Seven–Nine)

Field, Tiffany, Miguel Diego, Maria Hernandez-Reif, et al. "Tai Chi/Yoga Effects on Anxiety, Heart Rate, EEG, and Math Computations." *Complementary Therapies in Clinical Practice* 19, no. 4 (2013): 225–230.

Tsang, William W. N., Christina W. Y. Hui-Chan, and Simon N. Fu. "Effect of Tai Chi on Joint Proprioception and Neuromuscular Coordination." *Clinical Rehabilitation* 28, no. 6 (2014): 563–571.

World Health Organization. *World Report on Ageing and Health*. Geneva: WHO Press, 2015.

National Institute on Aging. *Falls and Older Adults*. Washington, DC: U.S. Department of Health and Human Services, 2020.

Harvard Medical School, Osher Center for Integrative Medicine. *Tai Chi and Health Outcomes*. Boston, 2021.

Safety, Ethics, and Scope of Practice (Chapters Eight & Ten)

Wayne, Peter M., David L. Berkowitz, Daniel E. Litrownik, Julie E. Buring, and Gloria Y. Yeh. "What Do We Really Know About the Safety of Tai Chi?" *Journal of Alternative and Complementary Medicine* 20, no. 3 (2014): 173–180.

Institute of Medicine. *Crossing the Quality Chasm: A New Health System for the 21st Century*. Washington, DC: National Academies Press, 2001.

Frank, Arthur W. *The Wounded Storyteller: Body, Illness, and Ethics*.

Chicago: University of Chicago Press, 2013.

Philosophical and Ethical Context

Merleau-Ponty, Maurice. *Phenomenology of Perception*. Translated by Donald A. Landes. London: Routledge, 2012.

Carel, Havi. *Illness: The Cry of the Flesh*. London: Routledge, 2016.

Levinas, Emmanuel. *Otherwise than Being, or Beyond Essence*. Translated by Alphonso Lingis. Pittsburgh: Duquesne University Press, 1998.

www.ingramcontent.com/pod-product-compliance
Lightning Source LLC
Chambersburg PA
CBHW070644030426
42337CB00020B/4160